CONTENTS

Ryan Cullenward a decorated Marine combat veteran & Lyndsay Ward a Bikini Athlete and Weight Loss Coach have spent the last 15 years helping others through health and fitness. More than just trainers but life long students of the science behind diet & exercise. Ryan has owned and operated nutrition stores helping formulate and sell products across the United States. He is a competitive nationally ranked bodybuilder as well as a bodybuilding coach & Lyndsay a weight loss coach, bikini competitor & designer together have led countless fitness classes and transformed the lives of their clients with their lifestyle program. TeamCully.com has a verity of program options to choose from plus a full contest-prep program for anyone looking to challenge themselves, get competitive, and live life on another level.

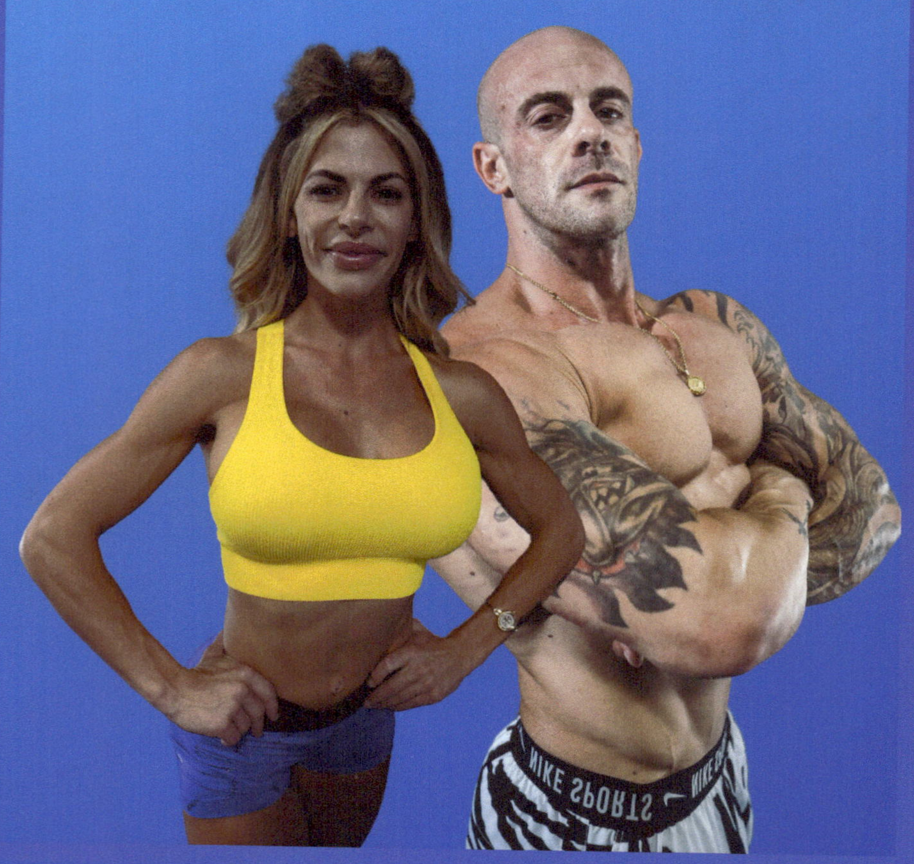

By making simple adjustments like your grocery list you can start to eliminate food you don't need and still feel full & satisfied.

Making these adjustments while following a carb cycle designed specifically for you, expect to start seeing major changes in how your body starts to develop.

Eliminating the food we love can almost always cause anxiety but in order to grow and make changes in our life the hardest things that need changing are usually the things that will lead us to success. Different food can cause humans to feel different states of mental clarity and overall happiness which is why it's so important to understand what exactly we put into our bodies and what those things do to us.

The great thing about carb cycling is you can still enjoy eating the things you love however understanding that there is a time and place. If done properly over a period of 8 weeks you can start to see results. Soon after that you will start to understand how to use food to your advantage with our carb cycling program.

Healthy ingredients & just the right amount of calories.

Almond Milk
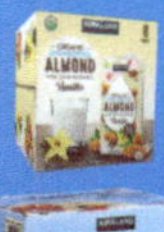

Egg Whites
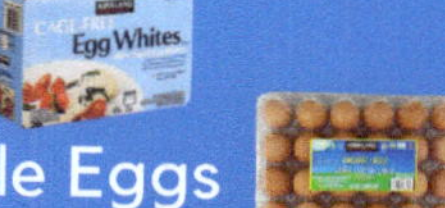

Regular Whole Eggs

Boneless Chicken Breast

(Frozen if preferred)

91% Ground Beef

(Frozen if preferred)

Mixed Veggies

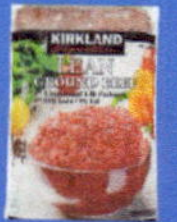

Quaker Oats
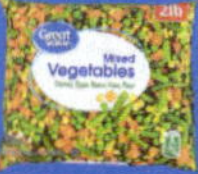

Krusteaz Pancake Mix
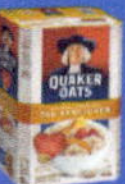

White Rice
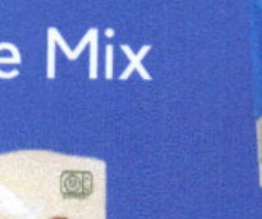
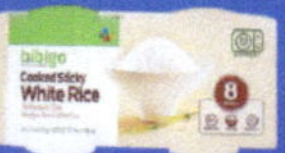

Natures Own Whole Grain Bread

Sweet Mesquite
(Seasoning)
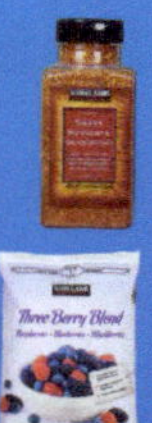

Dark Berries
(Frozen if preferred)

Strawberries
(Frozen if preferred)
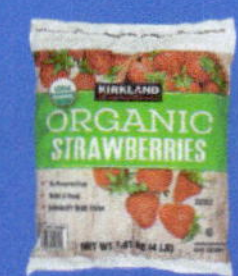

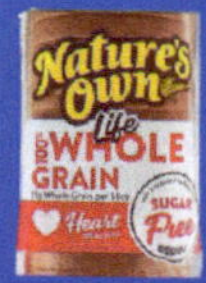

Client's who follow similar grocery lists.

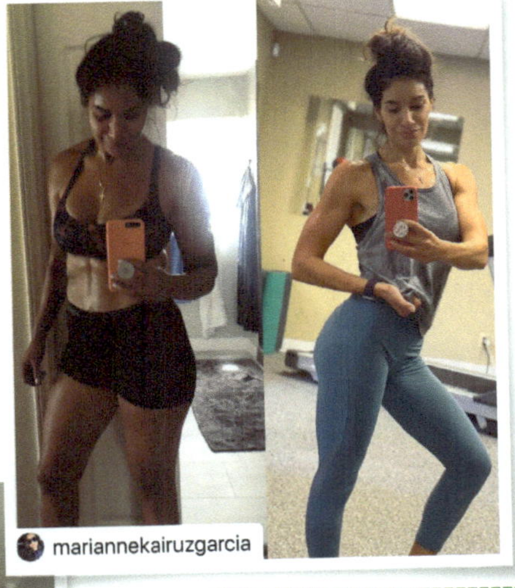

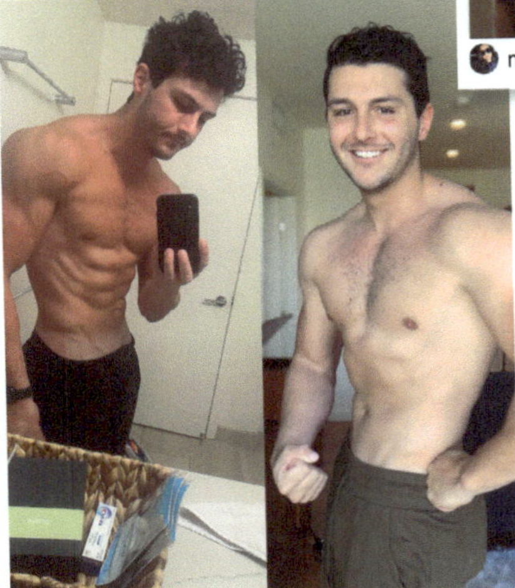

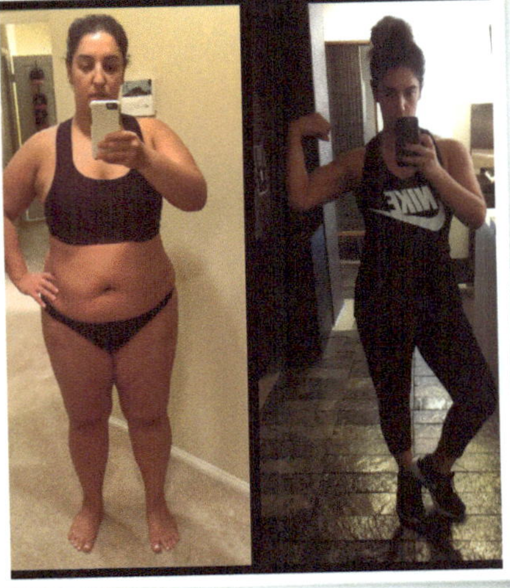

Our grocery lists are designed for efficiency & set up to get you into a solid routine for your monthly grocery shopping.

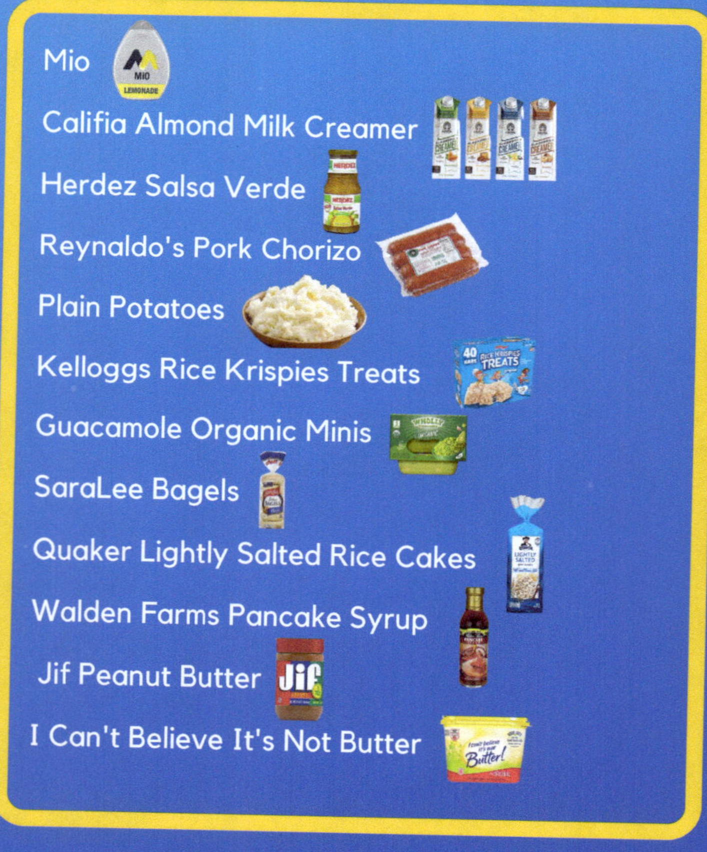

Mio

Califia Almond Milk Creamer

Herdez Salsa Verde

Reynaldo's Pork Chorizo

Plain Potatoes

Kelloggs Rice Krispies Treats

Guacamole Organic Minis

SaraLee Bagels

Quaker Lightly Salted Rice Cakes

Walden Farms Pancake Syrup

Jif Peanut Butter

I Can't Believe It's Not Butter

One of the most common mistakes people skip over is the use of condiments...sauce man.

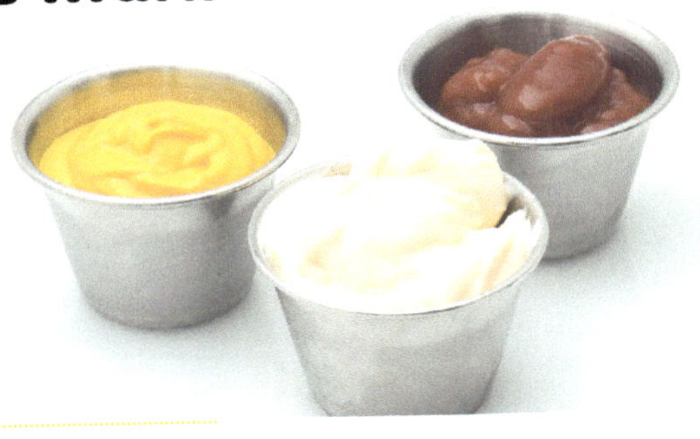

A lot of people don't realize that only a few serving sizes of any one of these basic condiments is your daily fat intake for the day. Why waste your daily fat on a few tablespoons of mayo when you could have had a donut or an extra serving of something more delicious?

Trying any new diet can be stressful and everyone deals with stress differently. If your like me I tend to eat and eat...and eat. It took a few tries to get on track, I had to start slow and ease into it. I live for food, it brings me happiness but I understood if I wanted to see change, I had to change. So I started by just removing all the basic condiments in both my fridge and pantry. I made this my focus for weeks 1 and 2 before adding in the next important variable.

Remove these basic condiments & try these instead

2 tbsp of any one of these can have up to 10g per fat per serving; or huge, dense amounts of sugar...this could be almost half of your daily intake.

Try this	Instead of this
I Can't Believe it's Not Butter	Butter
G Butter	Mayonnaise
Mio	Specialty Mustard
Coffee	Olive Oil
Salsa Verde	Ranch Dressing
Splenda	Syrup
Almond Milk	Creamer
Almond Milk Creamer	BBQ Sauce
Splenda Brown Sugar	Soda
Whole Eggs	Orange Juice
Walden Farms Pancake Syrup	Dairy
Chorizo (beef or pork)	Cheese
Lightly Salted Rice Cake	Honey

Dairy is scary learn to live with it.

If you're like me and struggle with things like depression, poor memory, anxiety, heart disease or overall mental clarity, dairy could be a contributing factor.

Why is dairy bad for humans?
Milk and other dairy products are the top source of saturated fat in the American diet, contributing to heart disease, type 2 diabetes, and Alzheimer's disease. Studies have also linked dairy to an increased risk of breast, ovarian, and prostate cancers.

**quality whey protein ISOLATE, will be lactose (dairy) free, due to filtering processes during production. Additionally, the proteins generally have the digestive enzyme (lactase) necessary to process lactose into glucose should you be lactose intolerant. Quality protein selection is key here.

Cully's Snack Hacks

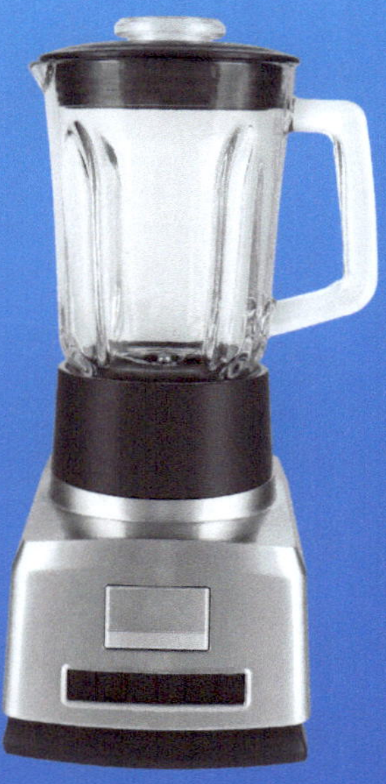

1 Scoop Titan Isolate Whey Protein
1/2 cup berries
1/3 cup almond milk
1/2 cup egg whites
1 spoon 16g peanut butter
add **4-5 ice cubes**

Protein | 40
Carbs | 12
Fats | 9
Total Cal | 289

Coach's Notes:

This is a great example of an easy smoothie recipe. The items selected are dense in specific MACRO VALUE, but not necessarily DYNAMIC in macro value. Making it easy to change the quantity of each item to suit your specific calorie or macro-nutrient needs.

It doesn't matter if you're on a lifystle program or prep .

A calorie is a calorie, a carb is a carb, fat is fat. You cannot change fact. If you program your carbs, protein & fats you can start to eat with intent & enjoy that burrito a little more knowing you're eating it for a purpose.

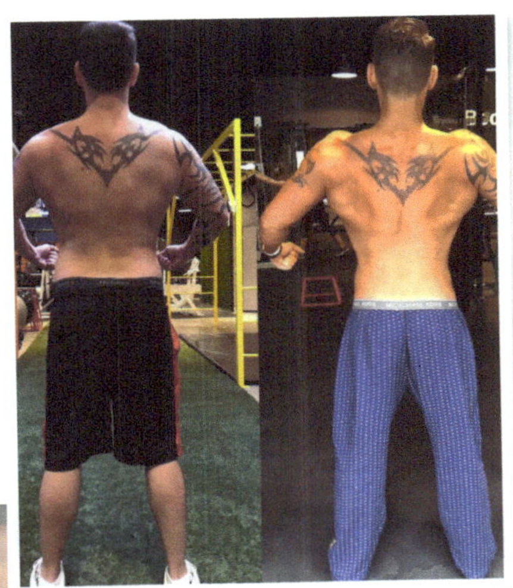

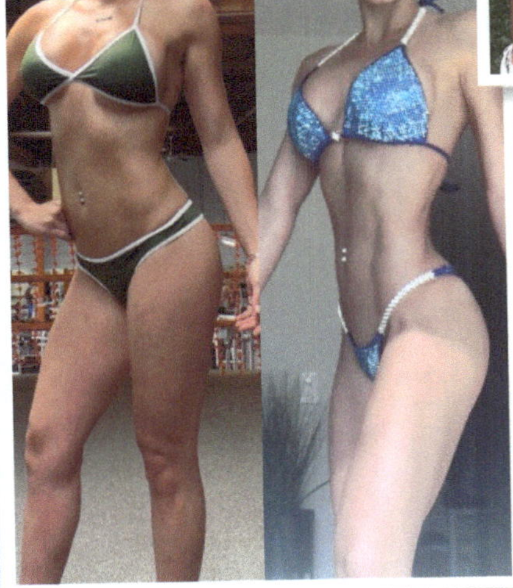

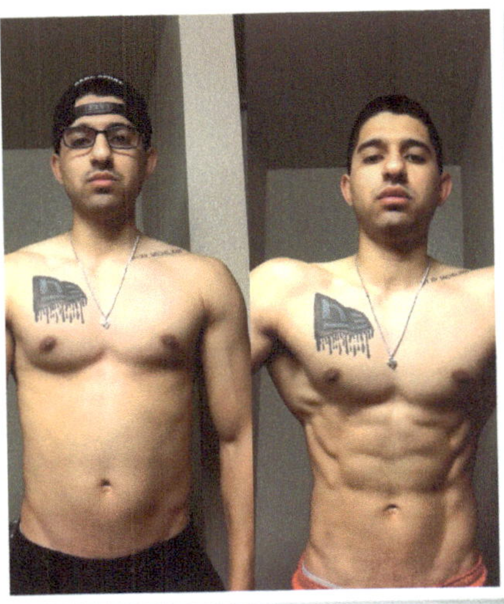

Cully's meal prep Hacks

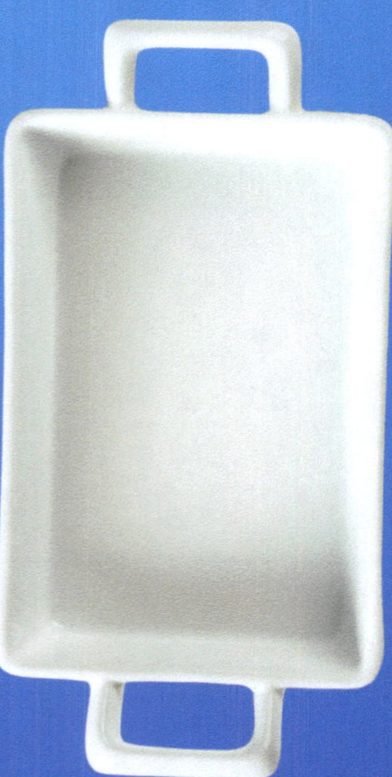

STEP 1

1 Cup - mixed veggies
16oz - 99% lean ground turkey
8oz -potato raw

Cook your meat & veggies first

STEP 2

Put mixed meat & veggies in baking pan
Cover top **with layer of mashed potatoes**
Bake **for 30 min at 350 degrees**

Protein | 104
Carbs | 50
Fats | 4
Total Cal | 652

Coach's Notes:

This is a great example of an easy to make, easy to prep and easy to pack meal, for on the go type people. It can be split into multiple servings, making those mid day meals easy. As long as it gets finished, you're golden . So if you can't get to a meal every 2-3 hours... NO WORRIES!!

You can use food to your advantage if you want to shape your body.

You don't have to starve yourself or go ham on the cardio. Our secret is structure, our programs provide structure so you can cruz & not hyper focus on your food, we got you.

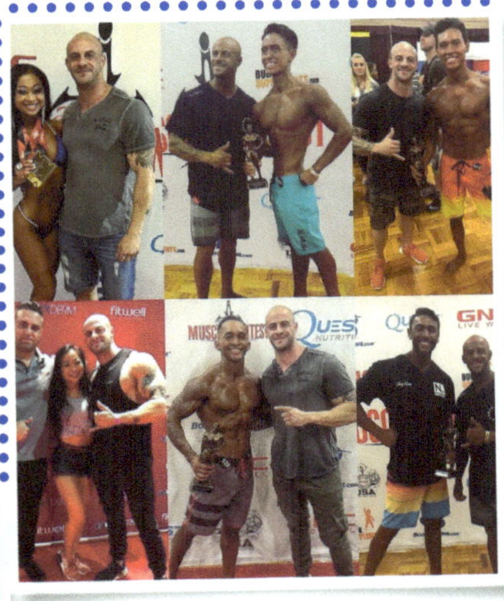

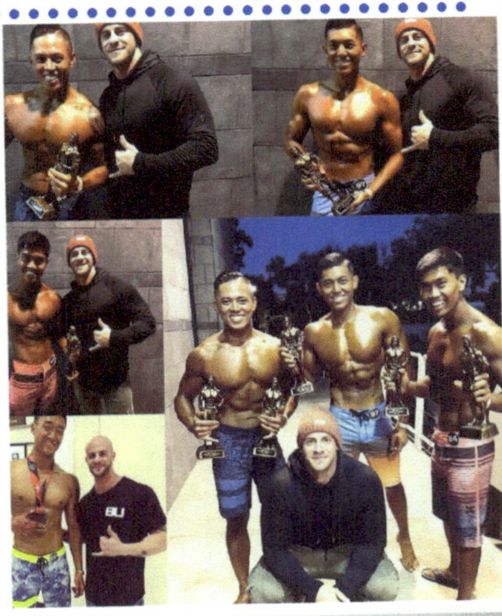

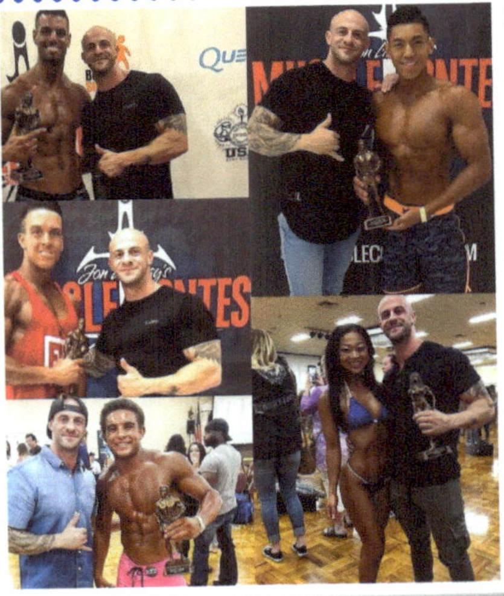

Cully's Snack Hacks

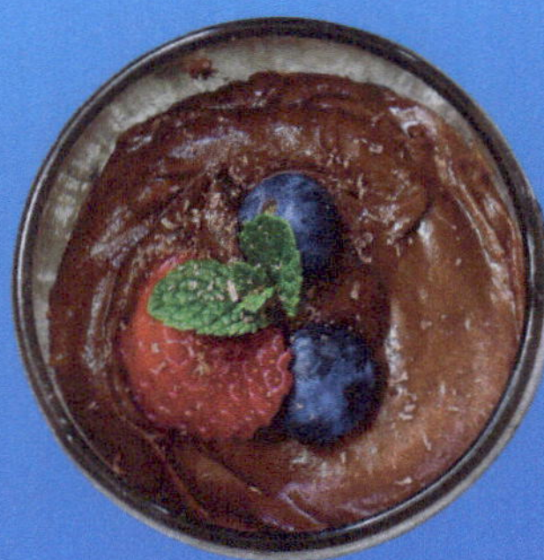

Cully's pudding

1 scoop - Titan Whey Isolate Protein

6oz - egg whites

1/2 cup - baby rice

*add almond milk if necessary

** Mix egg whites, little almond milk,and whey together; shake up and pour over the dry baby rice.

Protein | 43
Carbs | 24
Fats | 1
Total Cal | 277

Coach's Notes:

This is a fun hack that can be kind of like dessert, but remain very dense and effective as a meal. Add peanut butter to increase fats if necessary. Some times I like to garnish with a few sliced strawberries and some Redi-Whip, if i'm feeling sassy.

Combine food programming with exercise and anything is possible.

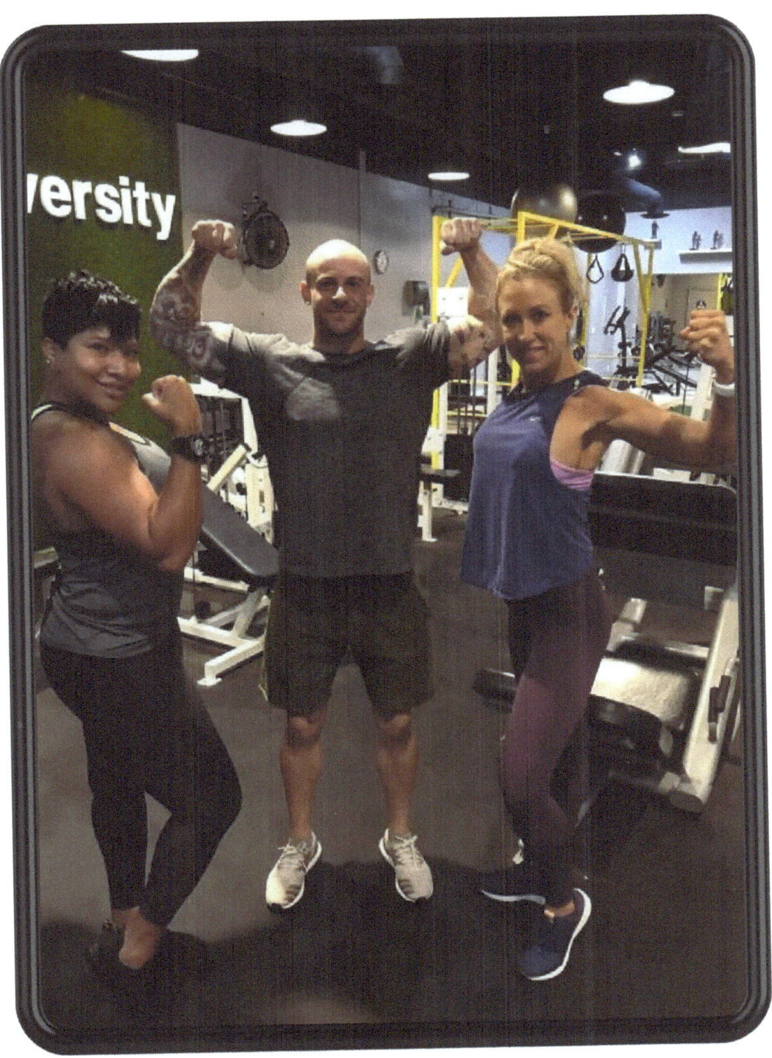

Cully's Snack Hacks

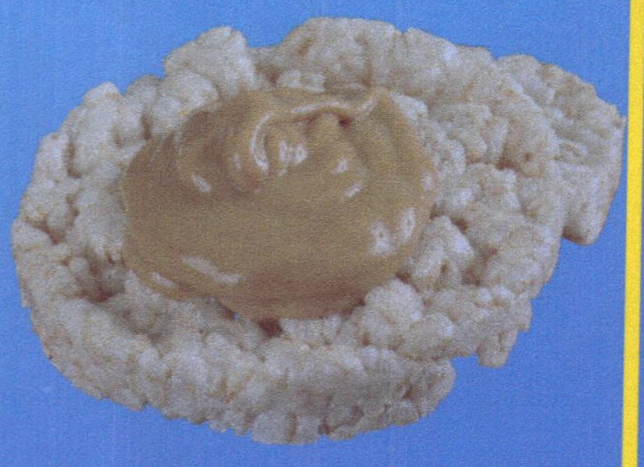

1 - lightly salted rice cake

16g or 1/2 serving -Jif Creamy Peanut Butter

**1 FULL SERVING - G Butter, instead of peanut butter, too increase protein a bit, and reduce fat. Perfect for those sugar cravings.

Protein | 3
Carbs | 10
Fats | 8
Total Cal | 124

Consistency is key

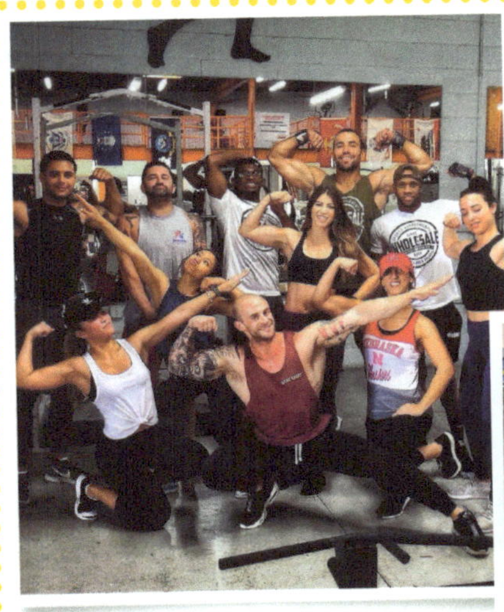

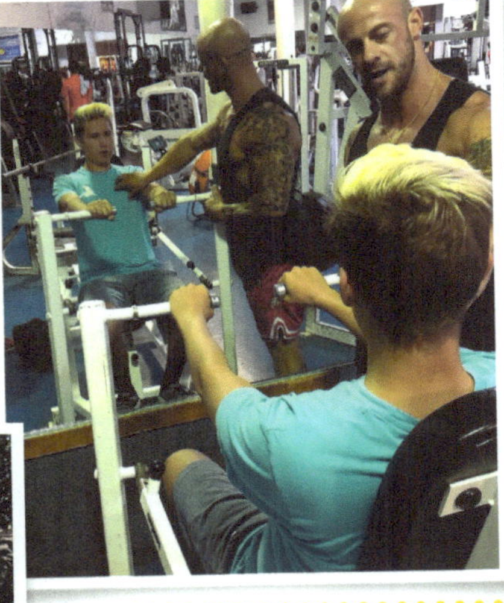

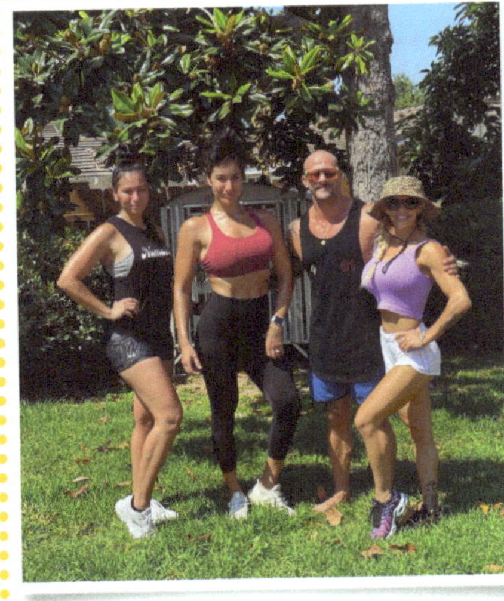

Cully's KEY to juicy meat!!

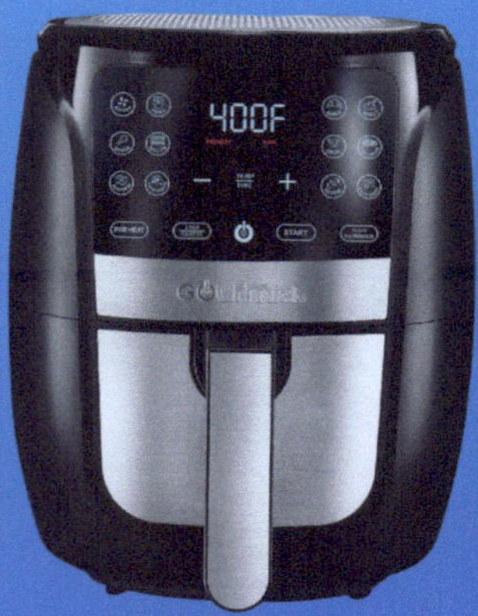

CostCo Deep Fryer
$56.99
Personal favorite prepare your meat & anything else in minutes!

Perfect for beef, chicken & fish.

The importance of carb timing while carb cycling.

The more we practice something the better we get, the same goes for eating. By following a monthly blueprint you can begin to understand that you can still enjoy things like donuts, sausage biscuits, pop tarts, waffles, hamburgers, etc. there's just a time and a place for it.

When you consume food try to start thinking of intent. Why am I eating, why am I eating this? Why should I take certain supplements before & after my workout? Can I be taking anything to improve my overall ability in everything I do ? What foods help my body grow? What level of intensity should my workouts be each day & how does that effect my food? How much cardio do I need to be doing with my daily food intake? When can I have a cheat meal? I messed up on my diet, how do I fix it?

It sounds like a lot to have to organize in your head but the more you do it the easier it gets. We believe that its 80% diet & 20% exercise, so if you hate working out there's a little bit of good news. But don't get it twisted, dieting is the hardest part. It will challenge you both mentally & physically. You will discover how we use food as a coping mechanism for everyday stress & life. By first recognizing what those tendencies are can we begin to work on them.

Sunday	Monday	Tuesday	Wednesday	Thursday	Friday	Saturday
	HIGH CARB LEG DAY • 30 minutes stairs • Have protein shake w/ donut after your workout	**1 LOW CARB BACK & BICEP DAY** • 30 minutes stairs • Higher fats	**2 LOW CARB ABS & PUSH UP DAY** • 30 minutes stairs • Higher fats	**3 HIGH CARB LEG DAY** • 30 minutes stairs • Have protein shake w/ donut after your workout	**4 LOW CARB SHOULDER DAY** • 20 min stairs • 20 min treadmill • Eat more protein if you get hungry	**5 LOW CARB CARDIO DAY** • 5 ROUNDS 25 Heavy dumbell squats • 40 minutes stairs
6 LOW CARB REST DAY	**7 HIGH CARB LEG DAY** • 30 minutes stairs • Have protein shake w/ donut after your workout	**8 LOW CARB BACK & BICEP DAY** • 30 minutes stairs • Higher fats	**9 LOW CARB ABS & PUSH UP DAY** • 30 minutes stairs • Higher fats	**10 HIGH CARB LEG DAY** • 30 minutes stairs • Have protein shake w/ donut after your workout	**11 LOW CARB SHOULDER DAY** • 30 min stairs • Eat more protein if you get hungry	**12 LOW CARB CARDIO DAY** • 5 ROUNDS 25 Heavy dumbell squats • 40 minutes stairs
13 LOW CARB REST DAY	**14 HIGH CARB LEG DAY** • 30 minutes stairs • Have protein shake w/ donut after your workout	**15 LOW CARB BACK & BICEP DAY** • 30 minutes stairs • Higher fats	**16 LOW CARB ABS & PUSH UP DAY** • 30 minutes stairs • Higher fats	**17 HIGH CARB LEG DAY** • 30 minutes stairs • Have protein shake w/ donut after your workout	**18 LOW CARB SHOULDER DAY** • 20 min stairs • 20 min treadmill • Eat more protein if you get hungry	**19 LOW CARB CARDIO DAY** • 5 ROUNDS 25 Heavy dumbell squats • 40 minutes stairs
20 LOW CARB REST DAY	**21 HIGH CARB LEG DAY** • 30 minutes stairs • Have protein shake w/ donut after your workout	**22 LOW CARB BACK & BICEP DAY** • 30 minutes stairs • Higher fats	**23 LOW CARB ABS & PUSH UP DAY** • 30 minutes stairs • Higher fats	**24 HIGH CARB LEG DAY** • 30 minutes stairs • Have protein shake w/ donut after your workout	**25 LOW CARB SHOULDER DAY** • 30 min stairs • Eat more protein if you get hungry	**26 LOW CARB CARDIO DAY** • 5 ROUNDS • 25 Heavy dumbell squats • 40 minutes stairs
27 LOW CARB REST DAY	**28 HIGH CARB LEG DAY** • 30 minutes stairs • Have protein shake w/ donut after your workout	**29 LOW CARB BACK & BICEP DAY** • 30 minutes stairs • Higher fats	**30 LOW CARB ABS & PUSH UP DAY** • 30 minutes stairs • Higher fats			
		o At least 30 minutes programed cardio o At least 50 minutes of weight training o 1 Gallon of water daily o No alcohol o At least 80% compliance of the program will determine success				

Always do your cardio after your workout for best results*

Exercise, it's important.

Like a lot of people, exercising is hard or finding the motivation even harder. Nonetheless in order to see results one must move their body if you want to shape it a certain way you can do that through carb cycling, structured workouts & cardio training.

Having your workouts timed around your eating schedule & overall life is important if you want to see maximum results. We can train & train but if we are not eating the right things around our training we will never see the results we are training for. The following is an intermediate/advanced training program for one of TeamCully's bikini athletes. It's easy to follow with exercises most people can do on their own in the gym or at home with the right equipment. If you think you need more hands on coaching we offer a more hands on coaching program with more communication, check ins & guidance. Check out our website for our other program options @ www.teamcully.com

ARMS

Hold & squeeze for a count, every rep.

EXERCISE	SETS	REPS
Shoulder Front Raise	4	15
Side Lateral Raises	4	15
Rear Delt Flys	4	20
Shoulder Presses	4	15
Barbell Curls, underhand	4	15
Tricep Extensions, rope	4	15
Machine Dips	3	20

ARMS
Track so you can program correctly.

EXERCISE	WEIGHT	REPS	NOTES
WEEK 1 1			
2			
3			
4			
5			
6			
WEEK 2			
1			
2			
3			
4			
5			
6			
WEEK 3			
1			
2			
3			
4			
5			
6			
WEEK 4			
1			
2			
3			
4			
5			
6			

After week 4 re-assess & go over areas that need improving, continue to track.

Back & Bicep

Hold & squeeze for a count, every rep.

EXERCISE	SETS	REPS
Lat Pull Down, over hand	4	15
Seated Row, cable or machine	4	12*
Bent Over Dumbbell Row, single arm	4	8-10**
Low Back Extension	3	15
Dumbbell Hammer Curls	4	10 each arm
Preacher Curls	4	15

*add a little each set, but not so much you cant finish the reps required.

**go as heavy as possible, add weight each set

BACK & BICEPS

Track so you can program correctly.

EXERCISE	WEIGHT	REPS	NOTES
WEEK 1 1			
2			
3			
4			
5			
6			
WEEK 2			
1			
2			
3			
4			
5			
6			
WEEK 3			
1			
2			
3			
4			
5			
6			
WEEK 4			
1			
2			
3			
4			
5			
6			

After week 4 re-assess & go over areas that need improving, continue to track.

Abs & Push Ups

Hold & squeeze for a count, every rep.

EXERCISE	SETS	REPS
Hanging Leg Raises	4	15
Decline Sit Ups	4	20
Cable Crunches	4	20
Standard Push Up	3	10
Incline Push Up, hands on bench or bar	3	15

ABS & PUSH UPS

Track so you can program correctly.

EXERCISE	WEIGHT	REPS	NOTES
WEEK 1 1			
2			
3			
4			
5			
6			
WEEK 2			
1			
2			
3			
4			
5			
6			
WEEK 3			
1			
2			
3			
4			
5			
6			
WEEK 4			
1			
2			
3			
4			
5			
6			

After week 4 re-assess & go over areas that need improving, continue to track.

Booty

Hold & squeeze for a count, every rep.

EXERCISE	SETS	REPS
Squats, wider than hip stance	4	12-15*
Hip Thrusts	4	12-15*
Reverse Lunges, smith machine	4	20 steps***
Hip Abductors	4	25
Deep Dumbbell Sumo Squats, feet on platforms or benches	4	10**
45 degree Glute Hinge	4	15

*add a little each set, but not so much you cant finish the reps required.

**go as heavy as possible, add weight each set

***20 total sets, 10 each leg. Can alternate or do consecutive one leg at a time.

BOOTY

Track so you can program correctly.

EXERCISE	WEIGHT	REPS	NOTES
WEEK 1 1			
2			
3			
4			
5			
6			
WEEK 2			
1			
2			
3			
4			
5			
6			
WEEK 3			
1			
2			
3			
4			
5			
6			
WEEK 4			
1			
2			
3			
4			
5			
6			

After week 4 re-assess & go over areas that need improving, continue to track.

Leg Day

Hold & squeeze for a count, every rep.

EXERCISE	SETS	REPS
Hammy Curls	4	15
Leg Extensions	4	15
Leg Press	4	10-12**
Walking Lunges, body or light weight	3	20 steps
Hack Squats	4	12-15*
Straight Leg Deads (RDL's)	4	15
Jump Squats, body weight	3	1 min

*add a little each set, but not so much you cant finish the reps required.

**go as heavy as possible, add weight each set

LEG DAY
Track so you can program correctly.

EXERCISE		WEIGHT	REPS	NOTES
WEEK 1	1			
	2			
	3			
	4			
	5			
	6			
WEEK 2				
	1			
	2			
	3			
	4			
	5			
	6			
WEEK 3				
	1			
	2			
	3			
	4			
	5			
	6			
WEEK 4				
	1			
	2			
	3			
	4			
	5			
	6			

After week 4 re-assess & go over areas that need improving, continue to track.

Essential supplements everyone should include in their daily routine.

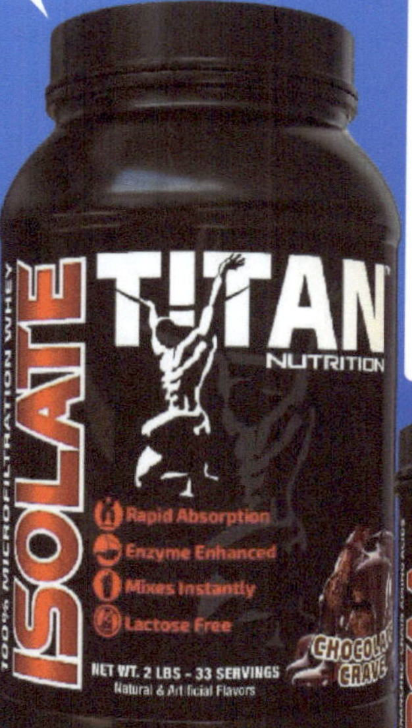

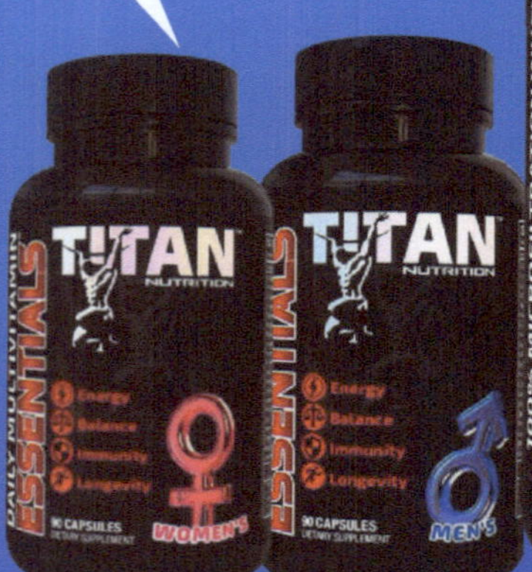

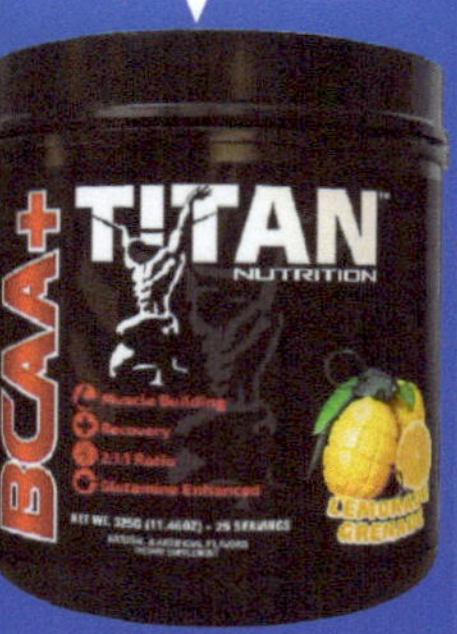

Titan Protein Isolate $59.99

Protein is essential for muscle growth.

Titan Essentials (men & women) $29.99

key to energy metabolism and nutrient breakdown.

Titan BCAA $44.99

Building blox for muscle.

All supplements available for purchase @ www.teamcully.com

You are what you eat

We aren't promoting eating donuts and just crap all the time....it's nearly an example of a, "not so clean" carb that can satisfy a craving, without derailing the plan. It's easy to calculate and not to crazy dense in added fat. Get some momentum before you start working in your craving killers. If you're focusing on cheats more than your goals, you're already losing!

Are all carb created equal? Well.. Yes and No. How carbs work in your body, how they are recognized, received, and the energy value per gram...? YES, all carbs are the same.

ON THE OTHER HAND
When it comes to things like Micro-Nutrient value, nutrient density, glycemic load values, and chemical responses on hormones in your body.... NO WAY!

If you need help

If you are not seeing the results you want & feel like you need help we offer a more hands on version of this program. Check-ins with coach, a meal plan that is specific to you, feedback throughout the duration of the program & the support you need to complete this course, it's ok to ask for help 619.988.8724